I0441643

FAST METABOLISM DIET

Boost Your Metabolism and
Achieve Lasting Weight Loss

The Secret of How To Eat
More Food and Lose More Weight

By

WaraWaran Roongruangsri

Part of the secret of success in life is to eat what you like and let the food fight it out inside.
Mark Twain

©Copyright 2014 by WaraWaran Roongruangsri - All rights reserved.

No part of this publication may be reproduced or distribute in any form or by means, electronic or mechanical, or stored in database or retrieval system without prior written from the publisher.

ISBN-13: 978-1514819142
ISBN-10: 1514819147

This document is geared towards providing exact and reliable information in regards to the topic and issue covered. The publication is sold with the idea that the publisher is not required to render accounting, officially permitted, or otherwise, qualified services. If advice is necessary, legal or professional, a practiced individual in the profession should be ordered.

From a Declaration of Principles which was accepted and approved equally by a Committee of the American Bar Association and a Committee of Publishers and Associations.

In no way is it legal to reproduce, duplicate, or transmit any part of this document in either electronic means or in printed format. Recording of this publication is strictly prohibited and any storage of this document is not allowed unless with written permission from the publisher.

All rights reserved.

The information provided herein is stated to be truthful and consistent, in that any liability, in terms of inattention or otherwise, by any usage or abuse of any policies, processes, or directions contained within is the solitary and utter responsibility of the recipient reader. Under no circumstances will any legal responsibility or blame be held against the publisher for any reparation, damages, or monetary loss due to the information herein, either directly or indirectly.

Respective authors own all copyrights not held by the publisher.

The information herein is offered for informational purposes solely, and is universal as so. The presentation of the information is without contract or any type of guarantee assurance.

The trademarks that are used are without any consent, and the publication of the trademark is without permission or backing by the trademark owner. All trademarks and brands within this book are for clarifying purposes only and are the owned by the owners themselves, not affiliated with this document.

Pawana© is a registered trademark of Pawana Publishing

Pawana book may be purchased for business or promotion use or for special sales. For information, please write to Pawana Publishing

Cover and interior design by Pawana Publishing

Interior photos ©Pawana

Author photo by Pawana Publishing

Author's Note:

I want to thank you and congratulate you for downloading the book, "Fast Metabolism Diet: Boost Your Metabolism and Achieve Lasting Weight Loss, The Secret of How to Eat More Food and Lose More Weight".

This book contains proven steps and strategies on how to boost your metabolism so you can still eat more of your favorite food without worrying that you will gain back all the weight you have lost. In fact, you will even lose more weight even as you eat more!

Therefore, the focus of this eBook is not on cutting back on, or eliminating entirely, some foods or food groups. Instead, emphasis will be placed on how you can boost your metabolism, shed those excess weights and, ultimately, keep them off!

If you take a look at many of the top models today, they give credit for their lean and slim bodies to their metabolism. Since they have fast metabolism, they have no trouble staying thin or staying in shape. But what about you, the lesser mortals? Does that mean you have to resign yourself to the fact that your metabolism is slow, and that you will never have a chance to lose weight and get the body you want?

Of course not. Although it is true that some of these people are born with innately fast metabolism, many more of them actually have to work hard at keeping their metabolism rate at a fast pace. Yes, it requires some work and a lot of discipline, and the Fast Metabolism Diet is an excellent example of that. For the time being, forget everything else that you have learned from the numerous weight loss trends and fad diets that have been introduced. It is time to get to know your body, be familiar with your metabolism, and work from there.

Be warned that the Fast Metabolism Diet is not a magic formula. Rather, it is a lifelong commitment, where you would have to make changes to your lifestyle and stick to it for the long haul. That is the only way that you can achieve the results you want.

Thanks again for downloading this book, I hope you enjoy it!

WaraWaran Roongruangsri

Table of Contents

CHAPTER 1
The Skinny on Metabolism

In school, we have learned about the different bodily processes, primarily digestion and excretion. We all have an idea how all the foods we consume are used by the body. We are even aware of the concept of the body "burning" the food that is eaten. However, not everyone has a full grasp on what this exactly entails.

This is the process called *metabolism.* This word is used to collectively describe all the chemical reactions that take place when the body attempts to maintain the living state of the cells. If we are going to be really technical about it, we can categorize *metabolism* into two:

- Anabolism, or the synthesis of all compounds that are needed by the cells to remain healthy. This promotes the growth of new cells, the repair of damaged cells and tissues, and the storage of energy for future use.

- Catabolism, or the breakdown of nutrient molecules in order to release energy.

From the above, we could simplify the definition of *metabolism* as the biochemical process of converting calories from the food you eat into energy that the body needs in order to function smoothly. In other words, it is the amount of energy (calories) that the body burns in order to maintain itself. The rate or speed of metabolism (also known as *metabolic rate*) is indicative of how fast the body converts all the food and drinks it takes in into energy.

How does this take place, you ask? Let us have a quick rundown of how it works. It starts with the intake of food. Food and drink that is chewed and swallowed undergo the process of digestion. The action of several digestive enzymes will break down these foods and drinks, converting them into forms that will be easily absorbed by the body. For instance, fats are broken down into fatty acids. Carbohydrates are converted into glucose, while protein is turned into amino acids, which are the building blocks of cells.

These will then be delivered to the cells through the bloodstream, where they will serve as energy supply for the cells and, ultimately, the body.

The Significance of Metabolism

The energy that your body feeds off on is courtesy of the chemical reactions involved in metabolism. The simple act of breathing or talking takes energy; the heart also requires energy in order for it to keep pumping, thereby ensuring that blood is supplied throughout the whole body.

In short, without metabolism, the body will shut down, and you are as good as dead.

The Variability of Metabolism

Have you ever wondered why some people have faster metabolism than others? In order to understand why metabolic rates vary among individuals, it is proper to first take note of the several factors that affect the rate of metabolism.

- Age.

  Children naturally have faster metabolic rates than adults. It is a fact that, as one grows older, their rate of metabolism slows down. For women, the slowdown starts once they reach the age of 30. This decline is much earlier than in the case of men, who will experience a slowing down of their metabolism when they are around 40 years old.

- Body Mass.

  This refers to the amount of muscles that a person has. The more lean muscle you have, the faster your metabolism will be. You can liken your muscles to a fireplace or furnace in your body, and they are responsible for burning the fuel or, in this context, the calories. It has been found that a pound of muscle can burn 40 to 50 calories per day. By adding more muscles, you will be able to burn more calories.

- Diet.

    There are specific foods that will aid your metabolic rate, while there are those that will simply slow it down. It is to be noted that this does not refer to the type of foods you eat, but also on the amount of food you take in, and the timing or scheduling of your meals. Eating at certain time intervals may also affect the rate that your body converts food into energy.

- Gender.

    It is another universal truth that men metabolize 10 to 15 percent faster than women, largely due to the amount of lean body mass present in males' bodies.

- Genetics.

    Sadly, heredity also plays a large part in one's metabolism. A person that comes from a family of people with fast metabolic rates is also likely to share the same trait.

- Hormones.

    There are specific hormones that take on the role of metabolizing certain nutrients into forms that will be easily used or absorbed by the body. This means that the body needs to continuously produce these hormones in order to ensure that metabolism continues. Disorders or other health issues that may cause hormonal imbalance will definitely directly impact the rate at which the food will be metabolized.

- Stress levels.

Emotions are also very influential when it comes to metabolism. You will notice that people who are subjected to high levels of stress are bound to have poor metabolism.

CHAPTER 2
Why Boost Metabolism?

We are now fully aware of the importance of metabolism and why we could not do away with it, or pretend that it does not exist. But is having knowledge about it enough? Is that all there is to it?

What many of us fail to recognize is why we should make sure that we boost our metabolism. Here, let us take a look at the reasons why we should take extra care in order to boost our metabolic rates.

Metabolism and Overall Health

Ultimately, we all want to be healthy - not to suffer from various ailments and diseases, and generally live longer - and the best way to make sure this happens is to place importance on our body functions. If all the cells, tissues and organs of the body are functioning properly, then we are guaranteed better health.

Metabolism ensures that the body functions in a more efficient manner. Therefore, the faster the rate of metabolism is the better. Having good skin, healthy hair, and looking great also go hand in hand with the body functioning as it should. You may have noticed this before, but people with faster metabolism are healthier, and they also look more vibrant and vigorous as they go about their daily routines!

Metabolism and Weight Loss

Metabolism has almost always been identified with weight loss, and this is not entirely wrong. After all, weight loss is the most obvious benefit of having a faster metabolism.

In order to lose weight, there are two things you can do with respect to your metabolism:

1. Eat fewer calories. This is so you can create an energy deficit, and there is less possibility that the food you eat will be stored as fats, or

2. Burn more calories from the food that is eaten. Keep in mind that, even when you are seated or lying down in bed, your body is already burning calories. Now, in order to burn more calories and consequently lose weight, you have to do more than sit down or lie in bed. You also have to increase your physical activity.

There are other perks of focusing on increasing your metabolic rate in order to lose weight.

- Unlike fad diets, the results are long term. This is because it addresses the *process*

(metabolism) and not the *tools* (i.e. supplements, lists of foods to avoid).

- You will be able to eat more without feeling guilty. After all, you have already come
to terms with your metabolic rate, and you
have also identified the manner with
which you will be boosting it to speed
things up.

Many are under the assumption that, in order to
lose weight, they have to cut back on some foods,
or even eliminate entire food groups from their
diet. But there are other advocates of "eat more to
lose weight", and they are those that believe that
focusing on boosting your metabolism is more
effective than completely redesigning, or paring
down, your diet.

It is also a fact that there are now a lot of food
supplements that claim to be able to increase
your metabolic rate, even if you do not exercise
or change your diet. They sound almost too good
to be true, and they probably are. Unfortunately,
many of these supplements also bring about side
effects such as headaches, dry mouth, and other
conditions that could potentially lead to more se-
rious health concerns and issues.

If you love food and your heart simply breaks at
the idea of giving up some of your favorite treats,
then you will definitely be relieved to know that
you can boost your metabolism, regardless of its

current rate. It is all a matter of training your body in order to have a faster or higher rate of metabolism, and that can be done in several ways! We will look into them in the next chapters.

CHAPTER 3
Boosting Metabolism
Through Eating Right

In order for metabolism to take place, you have to make sure you take in food. It is, after all, where the fuel that will be burnt through metabolism comes from. That is why the fast metabolism diet does not entirely rule out food groups. In fact, it even encourages you to eat in order for the body to have something to burn. While other diets discourage you from eating, this diet promotes it.

There is also the fact that you will be performing exercises in your bid to increase your metabolic rate. In order for you to be able to sustain performing those exercises, you need energy that will only come from food. You need to eat, and that is a fact that is acknowledged by this diet.

Eating right, in this context, means eating the right type of food, at the right amount, and at the right time. Follow this equation in order to succeed in boosting your metabolism.

Eating the Right Type of Food

Before we can proceed in naming the foods that you should eat and those that must be generally avoided, it is important to identify first the nutrients that you must focus on obtaining in aid to your fast metabolism diet.

- Carbohydrates

  If we are talking about "fuel", the first thing that comes to mind are carbohydrates. They are essential for building muscles and they are also the primary component of converting energy. The more you exercise, the more muscles will be built. The more muscles you have, the faster will be the rate of metabolism. Therefore, you have to increase your carbohydrate intake in order for the muscles to have an energy supply to burn calories.

  Other diets recommend that you cut back or completely eliminate carbohydrates from your meal plan. In this particular diet, however, it is recommended that 50% of your daily calorie intake should come from carbohydrates.

  When we speak of carbohydrates, we immediately think of grains and root crops. However, carbohydrates can also be derived from other, even plant, sources. Fibrous vegetables have fibers that aid in cleansing the body and ensuring the efficient functioning of the hormones and enzymes, as well as the cells, tissues and organs.

Examples of carbohydrate sources are milk, honey, grains and cereals (bran, brown rice, whole wheat, oats), root crops (potato, yam, taro), and fibrous vegetables (asparagus, broccoli, cauliflower, cabbage).

- Calcium

  Calcium does not only take care of your bones and teeth, they also help in muscle development. They are also contributory to the release of hormones that will, in turn, boost metabolism.

  Milk remains to be one of the best sources of calcium, although you can also get it from broccoli and other green leafy vegetables.

- Fats

  It is important to make a clear distinction between healthy fats and unhealthy fats. The fast metabolism diet advocates consumption of healthy fat in order to aid the action of certain hormones that aid in metabolism. In the case of other diets, they strictly prohibit the intake of any fat - good or bad.

  Of course, you also have to be mindful of the fats that you consume. The sources of good fats include avocado, olive oil, nuts, and sunflower seeds.

- Protein

  The cells' basic building blocks are the amino acids, and they are derived from proteins. Take note that it takes a long time for the body to break down proteins, resulting to a thermic effect to the body.

  Examples of protein sources include chicken breast, fish (salmon and tuna), eggs, milk, and whey.

What to Eat

Aside from the foods mentioned above, you should also include the following in your diet in order to speed up your rate of metabolism.

- Chicken is a good protein source, but focus on chicken breast or drumstick.

- Antioxidants are suggested by many, but the best antioxidant you can add to your diet is green tea. Not only does it have antioxidant benefits, it contains catechin, which is known to speed up metabolism. It also has the ability to increase the thermic effect of food.

- Fish rich in omega-3 fatty acids are effective in amping up metabolism, since they balance blood sugar as well as reduce inflammation. The best sources of these omega-3 fatty acids are herring, salmon and tuna.

- Add spices to your diet. The most highly recommended spices are cayenne and red hot chili pepper. They contain *capsaicin*, the component that brings that burning or hot sensation when it is eaten. This component can also raise metabolism up to 25% for a period of 3 hours.

- Soy protein has been found to be effective in boosting metabolism. Another benefit seen is how it aids in boosting one's immunity against diseases.

- Drink lots of water. Water remains to be the best cleansing agent of the body, ridding it of toxins, which is why drinking at least 8 glasses of water per day is highly recommended. Drinking water activates the process of thermogenesis, where the body will burn more calories in order to warm the water drank up to body temperature.

What to Avoid

- When eating chicken breast or drumsticks,

remove the skin. This is where the concentration of saturated fat and cholesterol is high.

- Too much caffeine can adversely affect metabolism. Go for alternatives that do not have as much caffeine, such as green tea and other teas.

- Cut back on junk food. Focus on healthy foods or, if it can't be helped, healthier alternatives to junk food.

- Ditch sugary soft drinks and soda. Instead, drink more water.

Eating The Right Amount of Food

In the fast metabolism diet, you are encouraged to eat more, instead of less. It is often called as the "eat more to burn more" ideology. This is so you can sustain the amount of fuel in your body as your metabolism goes to work. This is also partly the reason why you are actually urged to eat frequently throughout the day.

Eating frequently works by preventing you from snacking on unhealthy foods, such as chips and other processed foods, and will also prevent hunger pangs from settling in. If left unchecked, hunger pangs will force you to cave into the temptation of bingeing or overeating.

However, the main reason why you should eat more instead of less, is so that you will keep your metabolism going. Once there is nothing more to burn, metabolism will stop, and this is not a good thing, since your body needs to keep going in order for it to function properly.

It is like a machine. You should always keep it well-oiled so it can perform, and eating will definitely keep your body well-oiled.

Eating At The Right Time

Breakfast is the most important meal of the day. That is also a philosophy that is strongly supported by the Fast Metabolism Diet. In fact, it fosters eating early in order to boost metabolism.

When we speak of timing and eating, here are some tips that you should observe.

- Eating breakfast - especially a hearty one - will decrease the likelihood of getting hungry throughout the morning, or until lunch time. This will make it easier to resist the temptation of snacking at mid-morning.

  Oh, and do not skip breakfast. Often, those that skip breakfast end up bingeing in the middle of the day.

  It is also a good idea to eat your breakfast

early, so your metabolism will also start early. Eating breakfast late in the morning will give your metabolism a late start as well, and it is probable that you will proceed to eating lunch when your late breakfast has not yet been fully digested and metabolized.

- Snacking in between meals is not ruled out completely. In fact, it is recommended that you eat more than the usual three meals a day, and snacks are the best way to go about it. Try eating every 3 hours, which is just enough time for the thermic effect of food to take place.

  Ideally, men should have 6 meals a day, while women can stick to eating 5 times a day. Late night snacking is not recommended, however, since digestion slows down when you are asleep. That means that the food consumed during a late night snack will not be fully digested, and they will instead be stored as fat instead of being burned. Make it a habit to have your last meal of the day at least 2 hours and 30 minutes before bedtime.

- Since you are allowed to eat more than three meals a day, it is a given that skipping meals is a no-no. It is always advisable to keep a stash of snacks on hand, especially if you are always on the go and will not have enough time to sit down for a proper meal.

- When working out, it is a good idea to take a snack or meal that is rich with protein within 1 hour after your workout. Post-workout means muscle recovery, and that is best aided by adding protein to your diet.

The Truth About Calories

There is one rule that you should keep in mind when following the Fast Metabolism Diet: do not avoid calories.

Many dieters are extremely sensitive about the amount of calories that they take in a day, or per meal, for that matter. As much as possible, they choose foods that are low-calorie or even zero-calorie. It has its benefits, sure, but it is not really the best way to go about it. After all, calories are required for the metabolic process to take place.

Think about this: you are getting the right amount of exercise and you live an active lifestyle. Thus, your body needs 2500 calories a day in order for it to function properly.

But you are resolved to lose weight, and so you plan to limit your calorie intake. Instead of 2500 calories, you are limiting it only to 1000 calories.

That can't be good.

You see, your body is programmed, like a machine, to burn 2500 calories. However, there is only 1000 calories to burn. As a result, your metabolic rate will drop in order to keep pace with the calories that it is given to work with.

The result? You will feel more fatigued and out of energy, since the body has nothing to draw from in order to release that much needed energy.

Here comes another question: how much calorie intake should you have per day?

The answer will depend on several factors:

- Your age

- Your gender

- Your body type and size

- Your weight loss goals

More Tips to Eating Right

- Keep a food journal. This is the most effective way to keep track of what you ate, when you ate it, and how much of the food you ate.

- Be mindful of the nutritional facts of the food you ate. Read the labels. Find out what you can get from them, and how much you are getting. Pay extra attention to the calorie level, but do not fixate on it solely. Take note of the calories, but keep tabs on the nutrients as well.

CHAPTER 4
Boosting Metabolism Through Exercise

The key phrase here is "smart exercise". It has a marked difference with "hard or strenuous exercise", which seems to be the presumption by many. They think that, in order to speed up their metabolism, they have to pick the toughest and most demanding workouts or series of exercises.

That is not the case. So if you are thinking of re-working your workout regime to incorporate the toughest high intensity interval training (HIIT) or devoting more than three hours a day at the gym, you better think again.

You can easily rev up your metabolism without subjecting yourself to punishing workouts. In fact, you can achieve your goals with an exercise program that can be executed in short intervals, and with the least amount of effort.

Consider boosting your metabolism by incorporating two elements in your exercise program: *interval training* and *strength and resistance training*.

Interval Training

This type of training is characterized by performing high-intensity exercises and resting at specific intervals. It is also referred to as "metabolic burst" training, since the bursts of high intensity exercises are also the bursts of calorie-burning action that your body performs.

Compared to normal cardiovascular exercises such as running, biking or swimming, the objective of interval training is not endurance. After all, there are rest periods, and the whole interval training program can be as short as 30 minutes. Normal cardiovascular exercises can go on for a couple of hours or more.

Here is an example: pick a cardiovascular exercise, such as the mountain climber or the jumping jacks. Perform reps at the highest intensity that you can manage for a period of 20 seconds. Rest for 10 seconds. Next, perform the same reps at a lower intensity for another 20 seconds. Another 10-second rest. For the next 20 seconds, pick things up a notch and do the reps at high intensity. Rest for another 10 seconds, then perform another moderate intensity 20-second workout.

Here is another example: Run continuously for 5 minutes. Move to brisk walking for 2-3 minutes. This is considered your rest period. Then run again for another 5 minutes.

Take note that interval training requires periods of rests in between these bursts. This is to allow the body to eliminate the waste products that have been used in the exercise and subsequently stored in the muscles. When taking rests between sets, limit the rest period for a maximum of 45 seconds. That is the optimum rest period if you want to increase metabolism through interval training.

But you should also make a distinction between rest and "total rest". Some think that resting means completely coming to a stop and not doing anything. In those periods of rest, make sure you maintain even the smallest level of physical activity (e.g. marching or jogging in place, walking). This is to make sure that you keep the release of energy continuously.

Strength and Resistance Training

Your goal here is to build your body's strength and resistance in order to develop lean body mass or muscles. As mentioned earlier, having more muscles will boost your metabolism, and the safest and best way to build muscles is through strength and resistance training.

More than boosting metabolism, however, strength and resistance training also brings about other benefits, such as improved balance, enhanced flexibility, regulated blood pressure, and increased stamina.

There are many exercises that you can incorporate into your strength and resistance training regimen. That's the beauty of this program, because there is something for everybody.

- Strength exercises with weights

  Lifting weights is easily the most popular strength and resistance training exercise, largely due to the amount of tension that is applied to the muscles, depending on the weights involved. Continue lifting weights, adding more weight as your body adjusts and becomes more comfortable with the tension.

  One good thing about using weights in your strength and resistance training is how you can design your exercises to focus on specific areas of the body, or you can make it a full body workout, or targeting several muscles of the body. You can also easily adjust the level of exercise by making adjustments on the weights.

  There are some women who are apprehensive about lifting weights, thinking it would bulk them up. Keep in mind that the body of men and women differ, so their response to weight training will also be different. Women will develop muscles, but not the bulky kind that men develop.

  Strength exercises without weights

- Working with weights is not a requisite for strength and resistance trainings. You can also perform strength exercises and get great results even without weights. Examples of these exercises include the following:

  - Crunches. This is one of the most popular exercises that target the abdominals. There are several variations of the crunch, but it is important that it is performed properly to achieve positive results and avoid injury.

  - Push-ups. There are many variations to the push-up. One other exercise that is similar, and just as effective, is the plank. The plank also comes with variations, adding difficulty and intensity to the exercise.

  - Squats. The squat is a good exercise especially if you want to work various parts of the body, such as the gluts, the lower back, the hamstrings, and the quads.

Boost Your Metabolism Through Exercise

Determining which exercises to perform is not the only thing to pay attention to. You also have to consider the following:

- Level of intensity

  How many repetitions should you perform? How many sets? These are only two
  of the considerations you have to take into
  account when determining the level of intensity of your exercises. Of course, the determining factor or basis that you should
  use as your yardstick will be your level of
  tolerance. How far can you push yourself
  without overexerting it? You are the best
  judge of what your body can endure, and
  overdoing it will only be increasing the
  risks of injuries.

  When exercising, you should be able to
  feel the "burn" in your muscles. It is all
  right to feel some soreness and a little pain
  and discomfort. However, when your body
  is telling you that you are overtaxing yourself, and you are feeling signs of fatigue,
  you should pull back.

  According to the American College of
  Sports Medicine, the recommended level
  of intensity entails 3 or more sets of
  strength exercises, with 6 to 8 repetitions
  for each set.

- Duration

  It is possible that a person that spends 2
  hours a day working out at the gym still

has a lower metabolic rate than a person that does interval training for an hour every other day. This disproves the general impression that the longer your workout period is, the faster your metabolism will be.

When setting the duration of your exercises, it is important to balance that with the type of exercises and the level of intensity with which you are performing them. Consider this: a person exercises for 2 hours but only focuses on low intensity exercises with very long rests. Another works out for only 45 minutes, with high and moderate intensity interval exercises with 10- to 15-second rests. The latter is likely to succeed in speeding up their rate of metabolism than the first person.

- Frequency

You may know of some people that go to the gym or work out daily, while some are doing it only twice or thrice a week. Experts suggest that the ideal frequency of exercise would be doing them on alternate days of the week. The days in between will count as rest days. This is to give your body the time to recharge.

- Combinations

The best way to build muscles through exercise is by designing an exercise program that is essentially a combination of interval training and strength and resistance training – with and without weights. When choosing which exercises to incorporate into your program, choose those that will focus on the most number of muscle groups.

- Also, do not exclude cardiovascular exercise in your training.

When exercising, there is a huge chance that you will reach a plateau, and the amount of exercise you are currently having no longer has much of an effect to your metabolism. Kick it up a notch. Challenge yourself. Increase your intensity or even prolong the duration. This is why it is important to integrate interval training to your workout regimen.

CHAPTER 5
Boosting Metabolism
By Busting Stress

Stress and metabolism are inversely related. The higher your stress levels are, the slower your metabolic rate will be.

In this day and age, it is hard to stay stress-free. At every turn, there are situations that are potentially stressful. It is just a matter of handling the stress and not letting it get the best of you.

Stress has a particularly bad habit of affecting your overall health, not just your weight levels. Metabolism is where stress hits the hardest. If you are stressed, your rate of metabolism will visibly slow down.

Stress can also lead to the body producing more acid than it actually needs. It is important that the body maintains its 80:20 alkaline to acid balance. If acid goes up, the body's immunity is compromised, as well as the metabolism. After all, if you are sick too often, your body will not be able to handle performing metabolic processes.

Cortisol, the Metabolism-Stress Connector

Cortisol is a steroid hormone that is produced from cholesterol in the two adrenal glands that are located on top of each of the kidneys. Its vital roles include the following:

- Proper metabolism of glucose

- Regulation of blood pressure

- Regulation of insulin release to maintain blood sugar levels

- Boosts immunity

- Enhances inflammatory response

But cortisol is also popularly known by many as the "stress hormone", since it is secreted in higher levels when the body is in 'fight or flight' mode in response to stress. When cortisol is released, it offers the following positive changes in the body:

- It provides a quick burst of energy, putting the body in survival mode.

- It effectively improves memory functions.

- It enhances the body's immunity.

- It increases the body's resistance or tolerance to pain.

- It aids in maintaining homeostasis - the state in which variables are regulated, so that internal conditions remain stable and relatively constant - in the body.

But, as in most other things, too much will have negative effects. When too much cortisol is secreted, or when cortisol secretion is frequent as to be excessive, it can have negative effects, and they include the following:

- Suppressed thyroid function

- Imbalance in blood sugar levels

- High blood pressure

- Impaired cognitive performance, affecting one's memory and decision-making

- Decreased bone density

- Decrease in muscle tissue

- Weak immunity

- Increase storage of abdominal fat which, in turn, is indicative of health problems such as heart diseases and high levels of bad cholesterol, among others.

Dealing with Stress to Boost Metabolism

In order to deal with stress, you should focus on regulating and maintaining your cortisol levels. Doing this requires learning how to relax your body and eventually making lifestyle changes. Here are some of the most common relaxation and stress management techniques that you can employ to bust stress and, in the process, boost metabolism.

- Guided imagery

  Positive guided imagery is one of the simplest yet most effective tools in releasing tension and relieving stress. It can also provide insight and wisdom. The good thing about it is that, once you get the hang of it, you can do it pretty much anywhere at any time.

  So what does this involve? You can use tools such as an imagery tape, or ask someone to help guide you along. Or you could simply use your own imagination. It really depends on what you are most comfortable with.

  Call into mind or envision a very relaxing scene, and pay attention to its details, making all your senses work. You may also imagine someone asking questions about that better place, and you will have to answer all those questions, with one goal in mind: to get to that relaxing place, and stay there.

  Of course, not everyone can do it by themselves, which is why there is the option of approaching a professional therapist to guide you along. This comes at a price, though, so you have to be willing to spend some money if this is how you want to do it.

- Exercise

Believe it or not, some people find physical activity therapeutic. Some people practice yoga to relieve stress, while others bust out their running shoes and go for a sprint or a long jog in order to release some pent-up tension. For them, sweating is tantamount to de-stressing.

For those suffering from physical limitations, or those that cannot handle strenuous exercises, there are lighter options available. These include doing some gardening, cleaning the house, or doing household chores.

There is another exercise that many people tend to overlook: breathing exercises. Sit with back straight, close your eyes, take a deep, cleansing breath, hold it for 6 seconds, then exhale slowly. This is very simple, takes only a few minutes of your time, and it is completely free.

- Massage

How many times have you felt stressed out and gone for a massage session? Touch therapy helps in loosening tight muscles and joints, working out the kinks and knots brought on by tension. Getting a back or a shoulder massage works wonders. But if you have more time (and money) to spare, why not go for a full-body massage?

- Aromatherapy

  This is actually a good combination with massage. Essential and aromatic oils, when used in massages, provide a more relaxing effect. In some cases, the simple act of lighting aromatic candles in a closed room, turning down all the lights, and lying down on the bed, is already very relaxing by itself.

- Sound and Music Therapy

  There are people who find the sound of trickling water relaxing. Others even go as far as travel to the beach to hear the sound of the waves lapping against the shore or hitting the rocks. This is sound therapy. In many cases, however, music is their preferred option. They probably even have a specific musical genre or artist that they enjoy listening to and that helps them de-stress.

- Meditation

Through meditation, you are letting your body restore itself to a calm state, repairing it and bolstering it so it can prevent damage that may be brought on by stress. The key here is to let your breathing and heart rate slow down. It also aids in regulating your blood pressure, and the adrenal glands' cortisol production is slowed down significantly.

If you are thinking long-term, there are other methods you can employ in order to de-stress. Changing your lifestyle is highly recommended since, not only does it remove stress and boost your metabolism, it also promotes overall health and a longer and happier life. Here are some lifestyle changes and outlook tweaks that you should consider.

- Think positive thoughts. Get rid of negative thoughts and avoid letting feelings of negativity come over you. This stresses you out, clouds your judgment, and will likely make you do or say things that you will later regret.

  If you are going to think, think only of pleasant things. Do not open your mouth if you have nothing good to say.

  If you are having an attack of nerves, focus on calming yourself down. Try no to dwell too much on worst-case scenarios. Instead, try to think of ways to make sure you perform well on that presentation or on that speaking engagement. Visualize yourself doing well, and this will make you feel more confident as you go up the stage to do the actual thing.

Always worrying will undoubtedly cause indigestion. Some even succumb to nausea and flat out vomiting. There is nothing wrong with worrying, but if you let it overwhelm you, this will not be beneficial for you.

- Be consistent. If you decided to meditate in order to relieve yourself of stress, try to do it regularly. Meditating daily is highly advised. The same is true if you are turning to yoga for relaxation. Doing it for a week, stopping, and going back to it intermittently over the next several weeks and months, is not how it is supposed to be done. To get better results, keep things consistent.

- Learn to plan. Planning will take a load of things off your mind. Even the smallest activity, when planned well, will ensure that you will not be faced with unforeseen and potentially stressful situations. Avoiding stressors and stressful situations is considered to be one of the first steps to save you - and your metabolism.

CHAPTER 6
Boosting Metabolism Through Sleep

Sleep plays a crucial role in regulating one's metabolism. It is during sleep that the body is allowed to recover from the physical exertions it has been subjected to throughout the day. It is also during sleep that muscle growth takes place.

So what happens if you are deprived of sleep?

Sleep deprivation generally makes you tire easily, and the body will not have enough energy to sustain its workouts, or even simple physical activities. It is also possible that they will feel sleepy throughout the day, such that their productivity at work or at school will be adversely affected.

Sleep directly impacts various hormonal and metabolic processes in the body. It is the most important tool in maintaining the body's metabolic homeostasis. In terms of metabolism, the effects of sleep deprivation are more specific.

- Loss or lack of sleep causes an increase in cortisol levels in the blood. This means the body will be subjected to stress and the immunity is compromised.

- Glucose metabolism also slows down. If the person sleeps for extremely short bursts, glucose tolerance will considerably decrease, meaning the body will have a harder time managing blood sugar levels. This leads to higher risks for type 2 diabetes.

- There will be an increased difficulty in controlling one's appetite, resulting to overeating. This is because the hormones that are responsible for regulating the appetite will not be functioning properly, due to lack of sleep. Thus, food intake will significantly increase, and you will end up eating more than the calories required for your metabolism to work at the optimal rate.

So how can you boost your metabolism through sleep? It all boils down to taking steps in order to improve your sleep.

- As much as possible, try to get at least 8 hours of sleep every night. This is more than enough time to allow the body to fully recover and recharge for the next day. Although the duration of sleep will generally vary depending on some factors (e.g. age, gender, level of activity), it is still better to get more sleep than less.

- Sleep early. The normal circadian rhythm takes place from 10 at night to 6 in the morning. Therefore, try to sleep within that interval. Granted, circadian rhythms differ among people, but that is the most common period identified for muscle repair and renewal.

- Maintain a stable sleeping pattern. Having erratic sleeping habits hardly qualifies as quality sleep, so setting your internal clock to adhere to a sleep schedule is a good idea. Go to sleep at the same time every night in order to establish a pattern that your body can settle into.

- The sleeping environment also counts. Naturally, you want to sleep in a comfortable setting, since a fitful or restless sleep does not also count as quality sleep. As much as possible, make your bedroom conducive to sleeping. It is not a good idea to turn your bedroom into your workplace since you are likely to work instead of sleep when you are inside. Make it a point to emphasize the mental association between "sleep" and "bedroom".

- Stay away from alcohol, caffeine, nicotine, and other chemicals that interfere with sleep, especially when it is too close to bedtime. The stimulating effect of caffeine and other similar chemicals will prevent you from being able to sleep early.

- Do not force-sleep. You will only end up

having a headache if you force yourself to go to sleep. If you are having trouble falling asleep, do activities that will induce it. This includes reading a book or listening to soft music. Eventually, you will find yourself dozing off.

You may find the concept of "sleeping more to lose weight" a bit strange, but it definitely makes sense when you consider it with respect to metabolism. High quality and adequate sleep will put your body in a state that enables it to perform hormonal and metabolic processes. When metabolism is allowed to do its thing, you will have a faster and easier time losing weight.

CHAPTER 7
Metabolism and Permanent Weight Loss

Forget those fad diets that advocate starvation and 'eating less'. By focusing on your metabolism, you can still lose weight even as you continue enjoying eating.

Of course, it is understandable that one should worry how long the weight loss will last. That is the beauty of the Fast Metabolism diet. All the weight you lost through ensuring that you have a fast metabolic rate will not easily return, provided that you maintain a lifestyle that focuses on boosting your metabolism.

To cap it all off, here are what you should do in order to lose weight, and make it last!

- Eat right.

  Focus on your diet; eat the right types of food, at the right amount, and at the right time. Feed your body the calories that it needs to burn through the various metabolic processes. More than the other food groups, try to incorporate more protein and carbohydrates in your diet, since these two are the most active in metabolic processes. Of course, you should also make sure that you get enough supply of other nutrients, such calcium and healthy fats.

Timing should also be given importance when it comes to eating. Do not forget to eat breakfast and, as much as possible, have breakfast early during the day. Do not skip meals; instead, try eating 5 to 6 times a day, with an average of 3-hour intervals in between.

When working out, it is also important to eat after you have performed intense exercises. Have a meal or a snack within one hour after your workout to make the most of it.

- Exercise.

Maintain a certain level of physical activity, challenging yourself at every turn and increasing the intensity, duration and level of difficulty accordingly. Make sure to continue building muscles, or repairing them when they get damaged, because the more muscles you have, the faster will your body be able to burn calories.

Be smart about choosing what exercises you should perform. There is nothing wrong with picking those that target problem areas, but it is still a better idea to choose exercises that targets the most number of muscles at one time. Be con-sistent about your workout and stick to a schedule. However, make sure you allot rest days in between to allow your body to recover.

- De-Stress.

Keep stress at bay through various stress management techniques that you can do by yourself, or with the help of a profes-sional.

Sensation therapy such as massages, spa sessions, aromatherapy and music therapy are highly recommended, since they pro-mote long-term wellness.

You can also incorporate exercise into your de-stressing methods, and yoga is a perfect example of that. Meditation may take a lot of practice, but once you get the hang of it, it is a good way to relieve some tension at any time of the day that you need it.

However, prevention is still better than cure. Staying away from potentially stress-ful situations and always keeping a posi-tive outlook in life will definitely go a long way in ensuring that you remain in the best condition, and your metabolism along with it.

- Sleep.

    Sleep is still the best form of rest and re-covery that you can give yourself. No mat-ter how busy you get, you have to make it a point to sleep around 8 hours a day. Not only will this make your body recover, it will also revitalize it for the coming day ahead.

    You can compare sleep as a regulator, since getting enough of sleep will ensure that your body is able to manage its blood sugar levels. Metabolism will be faster, and you will also feel less tired during the day!

Conclusion

Thank you again for downloading this book!

I hope this book was able to help you to understand the principles behind the Fast Metabolism Diet and convince you that it is your best option to losing weight and keeping it off!

The topic on metabolism has always been a gray area for many, and how it relates to weight loss has proven to be an enigma. With this, we hope that you have gained a better understanding of the connection, and how paying attention to your metabolism is tantamount to putting an effort towards losing weight and managing it.

The next step is to assess where you are right now and apply these principles, so you can get the results you have always wanted in no time at all! The moment you become fully cognizant of the implications of metabolism to your quest for a lighter, slimmer, sexier, and healthier you, you will have no trouble achieving your goals.

So take care of your body and your health, and one way of doing that is to always keep your metabolism in mind. Eat right, exercise smart, bust stress, and get plenty of high quality sleep. With that, you are on your way to losing weight permanently!

Finally, if you enjoyed this book, then I'd like to ask you for a favor, would you be kind enough to leave a review for this book on Amazon? It'd be greatly appreciated!

Click here to leave a review for this book on Amazon!

Thank you and good luck!

WaraWaran Roongruangsri

www.ingramcontent.com/pod-product-compliance
Lightning Source LLC
Chambersburg PA
CBHW020905310526
45786CB00018B/1777